MAXWELL BENNETT

Top 50 Workouts: At Home Edition

Maximize Your Fitness with Minimal Equipment

This book was professionally typeset on Reedsy.
Find out more at reedsy.com

Contents

1

Introduction

Embarking on a Fitness Journey Right at Home

Welcome to "Top 50 Workouts: At Home Edition," your ultimate guide to achieving fitness goals without ever stepping foot in a gym. This book is crafted for those who seek to embrace a healthier, more active lifestyle from the comfort of their own home. Whether you're a busy professional, a stay-at-home parent, or someone who simply prefers the privacy and convenience of home workouts, this guide is designed to cater to your unique needs.

The Benefits of At-Home Workouts

At-home workouts offer a plethora of benefits. They are cost-effective, saving you from expensive gym memberships. They provide flexibility, allowing you to exercise on your own schedule without the hassle of commuting. Most importantly, they can be tailored to suit your personal fitness level and goals. Whether you're a beginner or an experienced athlete, these workouts can be adapted to challenge you appropriately and keep you engaged.

Principles for Effective Home Workouts

This book is grounded in key principles that ensure your at-home workouts are as effective as possible:

- Variety: To prevent plateaus and maintain interest, we incorporate a wide range of exercises targeting different muscle groups and fitness aspects.
- Progression: Each workout is designed to allow for progression in intensity and complexity, ensuring continuous improvement.
- Balance: We focus on creating a balanced approach that includes strength, flexibility, endurance, and balance training.
- Safety: Prioritizing safety, each exercise comes with detailed instructions and modifications to minimize the risk of injury.

Equipment Overview

One of the greatest advantages of at-home workouts is the minimal equipment requirement. While some exercises may suggest simple tools like resistance bands or dumbbells, many can be performed with just your body weight. We provide options and modifications for those with limited access to equipment.

Safety Measures and Injury Prevention

Safety is paramount. We'll guide you through proper form and technique to ensure that you perform each exercise effectively and safely. Additionally, we'll offer tips on how to listen to your body and recognize the difference between beneficial discomfort and harmful pain.

As you turn the page, get ready to dive into a diverse array of workouts. Whether your goal is to build strength, improve flexibility, enhance endurance, or simply maintain a healthy lifestyle, "Top 50 Workouts: At Home Edition" is here to guide you every step of the way. Let's embark on this fitness journey together, transforming your home into a sanctuary of health and well-being.

2

Warm-Up and Cool-Down

The Foundations of Every Workout

Importance of Warm-Up and Cool-Down

Every effective workout routine begins with a proper warm-up and ends with a thorough cool-down. These two elements are crucial for preparing your body for exercise and aiding in recovery afterward.

Warm-Ups: These exercises increase your heart rate, warm up your muscles, and prepare your body and mind for the physical activity to come. They reduce the risk of injury and can even improve your performance in the workout.

Cool-Downs: Post-exercise, cool-down exercises help in gradually lowering your heart rate and stretching the muscles you've just worked. This not only helps in recovery but also aids in reducing muscle soreness and stiffness.

Five Warm-Up Exercises

- Marching in Place (2 minutes)
- How to: Stand tall and march in place, bringing your knees up high.
- Benefit: Increases heart rate and warms up the lower body.
- Arm Circles (1 minute each direction)
- How to: Extend your arms to the sides and make small circles, gradually increasing the size.
- Benefit: Loosens the shoulders and prepares the upper body.
- Leg Swings (1 minute per leg)
- How to: Hold onto a wall for balance and swing one leg forward and back.
- Benefit: Warms up the hip flexors and leg muscles.
- Cat-Cow Stretch (2 minutes)
- How to: On all fours, alternate between arching your back and dipping it down.
- Benefit: Increases spine flexibility and prepares the core.
- Jogging in Place (2 minutes)
- How to: Jog lightly in place, keeping the pace moderate.
- Benefit: Boosts overall circulation and readies the body for more intense workouts.

Five Cool-Down Exercises

Walking (3 minutes)

- How to: Walk at a slow, steady pace to gradually lower heart rate.
- Benefit: Helps in transitioning the body to a resting state.

Toe Touches (2 minutes)

- How to: Stand and reach for your toes, holding the stretch.
- Benefit: Stretches the hamstrings and lower back.

Quadriceps Stretch (1 minute per leg)

- How to: While standing, pull one foot towards your buttocks and hold.
- Benefit: Stretches the front of the thigh.

Cross-Body Arm Stretch (1 minute per arm)

- How to: Bring one arm across your body and hold it with the other arm.
- Benefit: Stretches the shoulders and upper back.

Child's Pose (2 minutes)

- How to: Sit back on your heels with your arms stretched forward on the floor.
- Benefit: Relaxes the body and stretches the back and arms.

By incorporating these warm-up and cool-down exercises into your routine, you ensure a holistic and safe workout experience. They are easy to do, require no equipment, and are crucial for your overall fitness journey. As you progress through "Top 50 Workouts: At Home Edition," remember to start and end each session with these foundational exercises.

3

Full Body Workouts

Engaging Every Muscle Group

Introduction to Full Body Workouts

Full body workouts are an efficient way to exercise various muscle groups in a single session. These workouts are ideal for those with limited time, offering a balanced approach to strength, endurance, and flexibility. They can lead to significant improvements in overall fitness, metabolism, and body composition.

Ten Full Body Workouts

Bodyweight Squats (15 reps)

- Description: Stand with feet shoulder-width apart, bend knees, and lower your body as if sitting in a chair.
- Benefits: Targets quads, hamstrings, and glutes.
- Variations: Add jumps for intensity or use a chair for support if you're a beginner.

Push-Ups (10-15 reps)

- Description: Place hands on the ground, slightly wider than shoulder-width, and lower your body keeping a straight line.
- Benefits: Strengthens chest, shoulders, and triceps.
- Variations: Knee push-ups for beginners or decline push-ups for advanced users.

Plank (Hold for 30 seconds)

- Description: Hold the push-up position with forearms on the ground and body in a straight line.
- Benefits: Strengthens the core.
- Variations: Side plank for a different challenge.

Lunges (10 reps per leg)

- Description: Step forward with one leg and lower your hips until both knees are bent at about a 90-degree angle.
- Benefits: Works the thighs and glutes.
- Variations: Reverse lunges for a different angle.

Burpees (10 reps)

- Description: Start in a standing position, drop into a squat with hands on the ground, kick your feet back, do a quick push-up, and then jump up.
- Benefits: Full body exercise that improves strength and cardio.
- Variations: Skip the push-up or the jump for a simpler version.

Mountain Climbers (30 seconds)

- Description: From a plank position, alternate bringing your knees to your chest rapidly.
- Benefits: Works the core, shoulders, and legs.
- Variations: Slow down the pace for beginners.

Tricep Dips (15 reps)

- Description: Using a chair or a low table, lower your body off the edge, bending the elbows to a 90-degree angle.
- Benefits: Targets the triceps.
- Variations: Bend your knees to make it easier.

Leg Raises (15 reps)

- Description: Lie on your back, legs straight, and lift them towards the ceiling without bending the knees.
- Benefits: Strengthens the lower abdomen.
- Variations: Bend knees slightly if it's too challenging.

Supermans (15 reps)

- Description: Lie on your stomach and simultaneously lift your arms and legs off the ground.
- Benefits: Strengthens the lower back and improves posture.
- Variations: Lift only arms or legs for a lighter version.

Russian Twists (30 seconds)

- Description: Sit on the ground with knees bent, lean back slightly and twist your torso from side to side.
- Benefits: Targets the oblique muscles.

- Variations: Hold a weight for added difficulty or keep feet on the ground for stability.

Maximizing Full Body Workouts

For each exercise, focus on form over speed or reps. It's better to do fewer reps correctly than many with poor form. Listen to your body and adjust as needed. As you get stronger, increase the reps or duration, or try the advanced variations.

By incorporating these full body workouts into your routine, you engage in a comprehensive exercise regime that covers strength, endurance, and flexibility. Remember, consistency is key, and with each workout, you're a step closer to your fitness goals. Enjoy the journey and celebrate your progress!

4

Upper Body Workouts

Strengthening and Toning the Upper Body

I ntroduction to Upper Body Workouts

Focusing on the upper body is crucial for building strength, improving posture, and enhancing overall functional fitness. This section provides a variety of exercises targeting the chest, back, shoulders, arms, and core. These workouts can be done with minimal equipment and are suitable for all fitness levels.

Ten Upper Body Workouts

Standard Push-Ups (12-15 reps)

- Description: Place your hands shoulder-width apart and lower your body to the floor, then push back up.
- Benefits: Strengthens the chest, shoulders, and triceps.
- Modifications: Knee push-ups for beginners; elevate feet for a

challenge.

Chair Dips (10-15 reps)

- Description: Using a chair or bench, perform dips by lowering your body and pushing up.
- Benefits: Targets the triceps.
- Modifications: Bend your knees to reduce intensity.

Pike Push-Ups (8-10 reps)

- Description: Form an inverted V shape and perform push-ups, focusing on the shoulders.
- Benefits: Strengthens shoulders and upper back.
- Modifications: Lessen the bend for an easier version.

Arm Circles (30 seconds each direction)

- Description: Extend arms and make small circles, gradually increasing the size.
- Benefits: Tones the shoulders and improves joint mobility.
- Modifications: Adjust circle size and speed based on comfort.

Plank to Push-Up (10 reps)

- Description: Start in a plank, then push up into a push-up position and back down.
- Benefits: Works the core, chest, and arms.
- Modifications: Perform on knees if necessary.

Bent-Over Rows (12 reps each arm)

- Description: Using a dumbbell or a heavy book, bend forward slightly and pull the weight towards your chest.
- Benefits: Strengthens the back and biceps.
- Modifications: Use a lighter object for less intensity.

Bicep Curls (12 reps each arm)

- Description: With weights in hand, curl your arms up towards your shoulders.
- Benefits: Targets the biceps.
- Modifications: Perform without weights or with a resistance band.

Shoulder Press (12 reps)

- Description: Press weights or a resistance band upwards from shoulder height.
- Benefits: Strengthens the shoulders.
- Modifications: Use lighter weights or a band with less resistance.

Reverse Snow Angels (15 reps)

- Description: Lie face down and sweep your arms from your sides to overhead, like a snow angel.
- Benefits: Works the upper back and rear shoulders.
- Modifications: Perform without weights for a gentler exercise.

Side Plank with Arm Raise (30 seconds each side)

- Description: In a side plank position, raise your top arm towards the ceiling.
- Benefits: Strengthens the obliques, shoulders, and arms.

- Modifications: Perform with the lower knee on the ground for stability.

Tips for Upper Body Training

- Focus on Form: Ensure correct form to maximize benefits and prevent injury.
- Progressive Overload: Gradually increase the weight or reps as you get stronger.
- Balance: Work all parts of the upper body to avoid muscle imbalances.
- Rest and Recovery: Allow your muscles time to recover between workouts.

These upper body workouts provide a comprehensive approach to building strength and tone. Whether you're looking to enhance your physique, improve functional strength, or just stay healthy, these exercises can be a vital part of your fitness routine. Remember, consistency and dedication are key to seeing results. Happy training!

5

Lower Body Workouts

Building Strength and Endurance in the Lower Body

Introduction to Lower Body Workouts

The lower body contains some of the largest muscles in our body, crucial for everyday movements, balance, and overall strength. This section focuses on exercises targeting the thighs, glutes, calves, and hamstrings. These workouts can be performed at home with no or minimal equipment and are suitable for various fitness levels.

Ten Lower Body Workouts

Bodyweight Squats (15-20 reps)

- Description: Stand with feet shoulder-width apart and squat down as if sitting back in a chair.

- Benefits: Engages quads, hamstrings, and glutes.
- Adaptations: Use a chair for support or add a jump for intensity.

Lunges (12 reps per leg)

- Description: Step forward into a lunge position, ensuring your knee doesn't go over your toe.
- Benefits: Works the thighs and glutes.
- Adaptations: Reverse lunges or walking lunges for variety.

Calf Raises (20 reps)

- Description: Stand on the edge of a step and raise your heels, then lower them below the step level.
- Benefits: Strengthens the calf muscles.
- Adaptations: Do one leg at a time for added difficulty.

Glute Bridges (15 reps)

- Description: Lie on your back with knees bent and lift your hips off the ground.
- Benefits: Targets the glutes and lower back.
- Adaptations: Single-leg bridge for a challenge.

Side Leg Raises (15 reps each side)

- Description: Lie on your side and lift the upper leg up and down in a controlled manner.
- Benefits: Works the outer thighs and glutes.
- Adaptations: Add ankle weights for more resistance.

Donkey Kicks (15 reps each leg)

- Description: On all fours, kick one leg back and up, keeping your knee bent.
- Benefits: Strengthens glutes and hamstrings.
- Adaptations: Add resistance with a band or ankle weights.

Sumo Squats (15 reps)

- Description: Stand with feet wider than shoulder-width and toes pointing out, then squat.
- Benefits: Targets inner thighs and glutes.
- Adaptations: Hold a weight for added resistance.

Step-Ups (15 reps each leg)

- Description: Step up onto a sturdy chair or bench, then step back down.
- Benefits: Works the thighs and glutes.
- Adaptations: Add a knee raise for more intensity.

Wall Sit (Hold for 30-60 seconds)

- Description: Lean against a wall and slide down into a seated position, holding the pose.
- Benefits: Strengthens quads and improves endurance.
- Adaptations: Hold a weight for added challenge.

Single-Leg Deadlifts (12 reps each leg)

- Description: Stand on one leg and lean forward, reaching towards

the ground, and then return to standing.
- Benefits: Engages hamstrings and improves balance.
- Adaptations: Hold a dumbbell for added resistance.

Maximizing Lower Body Workouts

- Ensure proper form to prevent injuries and maximize benefits.
- Focus on controlled movements to engage the muscles effectively.
- Gradually increase repetitions or add weights as you progress.
- Allow adequate rest between workouts for muscle recovery.

These lower body exercises offer a comprehensive approach to strengthening and toning your lower body. They can improve your functional strength, enhance your body shape, and increase your overall fitness levels. Consistent effort and gradual progression are key to achieving the best results from these workouts.

6

Core and Stability Workouts

Enhancing Core Strength and Balance

Introduction to Core and Stability Workouts

A strong core is essential for overall body strength, balance, and posture. Core workouts target not just the abdominal muscles, but also the muscles around your pelvis, lower back, and hips. Stability exercises improve your balance and coordination, which is crucial for both everyday activities and athletic performance. This section focuses on exercises that build core strength and enhance stability, suitable for a range of fitness levels and requiring minimal equipment.

Ten Core and Stability Workouts

Plank (Hold for 30-60 seconds)

- Description: Maintain a push-up position with forearms on the ground, body in a straight line.

19

- Benefits: Strengthens the entire core.
- Adjustments: Plank on knees for beginners or add leg lifts for a challenge.

Russian Twists (20 reps)

- Description: Sit on the floor, lean back slightly, lift feet, and twist the torso side to side.
- Benefits: Targets obliques and rotational strength.
- Adjustments: Keep feet on the ground for stability or hold a weight for added difficulty.

Bicycle Crunches (20 reps)

- Description: Lie on your back, bring your knees in towards your chest, and alternate touching your elbows to the opposite knee.
- Benefits: Works the entire abdominal region.
- Adjustments: Slow down the motion for better control.

Leg Raises (15 reps)

- Description: Lie on your back, keep legs straight, and raise them up and down without touching the floor.
- Benefits: Strengthens lower abdominals.
- Adjustments: Bend knees slightly to reduce intensity.

Side Plank (30 seconds each side)

- Description: Lie on your side, prop yourself up on one forearm and stack your feet, lifting your hips.
- Benefits: Strengthens obliques and improves lateral stability.

- Adjustments: Lower the bottom knee to the ground for support.

Bird Dog (15 reps each side)

- Description: On all fours, extend one arm and the opposite leg, then switch sides.
- Benefits: Improves core stability and balance.
- Adjustments: Raise only an arm or leg if extending both is too challenging.

Dead Bug (15 reps)

- Description: Lie on your back, arms extended towards the ceiling, and alternate extending opposite arm and leg.
- Benefits: Enhances core stability and coordination.
- Adjustments: Move slower for more control or only extend one limb at a time.

Flutter Kicks (30 seconds)

- Description: Lie on your back, lift your legs slightly, and kick them up and down in a small, rapid motion.
- Benefits: Targets lower abs and hip flexors.
- Adjustments: Place hands under hips for lower back support.

Mountain Climbers (30 seconds)

- Description: From a plank position, rapidly bring your knees towards your chest.
- Benefits: Works the core and improves cardiovascular fitness.
- Adjustments: Slow the pace to focus more on stability.

Reverse Crunches (15 reps)

- Description: Lie on your back, lift your knees towards your chest, and curl your hips off the floor.
- Benefits: Targets the lower abdominals.
- Adjustments: Perform with a slower motion for better muscle engagement.

Tips for Core and Stability Training

- Focus on Quality: Prioritize proper form and controlled movements over the number of repetitions.
- Breathe: Proper breathing is crucial for core exercises to maximize effectiveness.
- Consistency: Regularly include these exercises in your routine for the best results.
- Progression: As you get stronger, increase the duration or reps, or try more challenging variations.

These core and stability exercises are designed to build a strong foundation for your body, improving your posture, balance, and overall fitness. Integrating these exercises into your workout routine will not only enhance your physical appearance but also contribute significantly to your functional strength and injury prevention. Stay committed, and enjoy the journey to a stronger, more stable you!

7

Cardio Workouts

Boosting Cardiovascular Health at Home

Importance of Cardiovascular Health

Cardiovascular exercises are essential for improving heart health, increasing stamina, and aiding in weight loss. They also play a significant role in reducing the risk of many chronic diseases. At-home cardio workouts can be just as effective as outdoor or gym-based cardio exercises. This section introduces five simple yet effective cardio workouts that can be performed in the comfort of your home, suitable for all fitness levels.

Five Effective Cardio Workouts at Home

Jumping Jacks (3 sets of 1 minute)

- Description: Stand straight, then jump with legs spread and hands touching overhead.

- Benefits: Increases heart rate, improves coordination and stamina.
- Adaptation: Step side to side instead of jumping for a low-impact version.

High Knees (3 sets of 45 seconds)

- Description: Jog in place, bringing your knees as high as possible.
- Benefits: Enhances cardiovascular endurance and engages core muscles.
- Adaptation: March in place with high knees for a lower impact.

Burpees (3 sets of 10 reps)

- Description: Start in a standing position, drop into a squat with hands on the ground, kick your feet back, do a push-up, and jump up.
- Benefits: Full-body exercise that improves strength and cardio.
- Adaptation: Remove the jump and/or push-up for less intensity.

Skater Jumps (3 sets of 30 seconds)

- Description: Leap from side to side, landing on one foot like a speed skater.
- Benefits: Improves lateral movement, balance, and cardiovascular health.
- Adaptation: Step instead of jump for a lower impact option.

Mountain Climbers (3 sets of 30 seconds)

- Description: From a plank position, alternate bringing your knees to your chest rapidly.

- Benefits: Strengthens the core and increases heart rate.
- Adaptation: Slow down the pace for a more controlled, less intense workout.

Maximizing Cardio Workouts at Home

- Stay Hydrated: Cardio exercises increase sweating, so drink plenty of water.
- Warm-Up: Always start with a warm-up to prepare your body and prevent injuries.
- Consistency: Regular cardio workouts are key to improving cardiovascular health.
- Space: Ensure you have enough space to move safely without any obstacles.

These cardio exercises are designed to raise your heart rate, burn calories, and boost your overall health. They can be easily modified to suit your fitness level and space constraints. Remember, the key to cardiovascular fitness is regular and consistent exercise, so try to incorporate these activities into your weekly routine for optimal health benefits.

8

Appendices for "Top 50 Workouts: At Home Edition"

Appendix 1: Workout Schedules for Different Goals

1. Weight Loss Focus

- A 4-week plan emphasizing cardio and high-rep, low-weight strength training.

2. Muscle Building Focus

- A 6-week plan focusing on progressive overload and strength training with adequate rest.

3. General Fitness and Well-being

- A continuous, adaptable plan for those looking to maintain health and fitness.

4. Flexibility and Mobility Focus

- A plan incorporating yoga, stretching, and mobility exercises.

Appendix 2: Nutritional Tips to Complement Workouts

1. Balanced Diet Fundamentals

- Overview of a healthy, balanced diet and its importance in fitness.

2. Pre and Post-Workout Nutrition

- Suggestions for optimal foods and timing to maximize workout benefits.

3. Hydration

- Guidelines on water intake before, during, and after workouts.

4. Supplements

- An overview of common supplements and their potential benefits and risks.

Appendix 3: References and Further Reading

1. Exercise Physiology and Anatomy

- A list of resources for those interested in understanding the science behind the exercises.

2. Nutritional Science

- Recommended readings on nutrition for fitness and health.

3. Mind-Body Connection

- Resources on the importance of mental health in physical fitness.

4. Advanced Training Techniques

- For readers who wish to delve deeper into specialized training methods.

These appendices are designed to provide additional support and information to help you on your fitness journey. Whether your goal is to lose weight, build muscle, enhance flexibility, or simply maintain a healthy lifestyle, the right combination of workouts and nutrition is key. The resources and plans outlined here can be adapted to suit individual needs and preferences, ensuring a holistic approach to health and wellness.

9

Resources

Recommended Websites and Online Resources

- FitnessBlender.com
- A comprehensive resource offering a variety of at-home workout videos and fitness tips.
- Darebee.com
- Provides a wide range of fitness routines, including bodyweight exercises and challenges.
- YogaWithAdriene.com
- Offers free yoga videos suitable for all levels, focusing on flexibility and mindfulness.
- MyFitnessPal.com
- A tool for tracking diet and exercise, and accessing a large community for support and advice.
- ExRx.net
- A detailed resource for exercise instruction, anatomy, and kinesiology.

Recommended Books

- "Body by You" by Mark Lauren
- Focuses on bodyweight exercises and creating personalized workout routines.
- "The Women's Health Big Book of Exercises" by Adam Campbell
- Offers a variety of exercises and workout plans, with a focus on female fitness.
- "Bigger Leaner Stronger" by Michael Matthews
- A guide to building muscle, losing fat, and getting healthy without a gym.
- "Yoga Anatomy" by Leslie Kaminoff and Amy Matthews
- Provides an in-depth look at yoga poses and the anatomy involved.

Podcasts for Fitness Enthusiasts

- The Dumbbells
- A comedic fitness podcast where hosts discuss health, fitness, and answer questions.
- The Mind Pump Podcast
- Fitness experts delve into health, fitness, nutrition, and more.
- Iron Radio
- Focuses on topics around bodybuilding, powerlifting, and health.

YouTube Channels

- Fitness Blender
- Offers a variety of workout videos, from HIIT to strength training, suitable for all levels.
- POPSUGAR Fitness
- Provides fun and trendy fitness tutorials, workouts, and fitness tips.

- Athlean-X
- Hosted by physical therapist and strength coach Jeff Cavaliere, focusing on training and nutrition.